SURVIVING BRAIN CANCER:

How To Deal With Brain Cancer

Dr. Bobby Franklin

DEDICATION

This book is dedicated to people battling cancer and to those who have died from this deadly illness. My thoughts are with their families and loved ones. Together we can win this battle against cancer.

TABLE OF CONTENT

CHAPTER 1

DEFINITION OF BRAIN CANCER

Brain cancer, additionally regarded as a brain tumor, can be defined as the strange increase of cells in the brain or its surrounding tissues. Brain cancer can be primary, in which skill originates in the brain, or secondary, in which potential it has spread to the brain from different parts of the body.

There are many exclusive kinds of brain cancer, every with special characteristics and treatment options. Some brain tumors are benign, meaning they do not unfold to different parts of the physique and can often be efficiently treated with a surgical operation or different therapies. However, other brain tumors are malignant, in which capacity they can unfold to different parts of the brain or physique and require greater aggressive treatments, such as chemotherapy or radiation therapy.

A brain tumor is a growth of odd cells in the brain. The anatomy of the brain is very complex, with exclusive components accountable for different apprehensive device functions. Brain tumors can increase in any part of the brain or skull, inclusive of its shielding lining, the underside of the brain (skull base), the brainstem, the sinuses and the nasal cavity, and many different areas. There are extra than 120 unique kinds of tumors that can advance in the brain, depending on what tissue they occur from.

How Common Are brain Tumors, And Are They Dangerous?
In the United States, Brain and fearful system tumors affect about 30 adults out of 100,000. Brain tumors are dangerous because they can put a strain on healthful parts of the brain or spread into those areas. Some brain tumors can additionally be cancerous or grow to be cancerous. They can cause trouble if they block

the flow of fluid around the brain, which can lead to an enlargement in stress inner the skull. Some sorts of tumors can unfold through the spinal fluid to distant areas of the brain or the spine.

How Is A Tumor Different From A Brain Lesion?

A Brain tumor is a unique type of brain lesion. A lesion describes any region of damaged tissue. All tumors are lesions, however, now not all lesions are tumors. Other brain lesions can be triggered through stroke, injury, encephalitis, and arteriovenous malformation.

Brain Tumor Vs. Brain Lesion

All brain cancers are tumors, however, not all brain tumors are cancerous. Noncancerous brain tumors are known as benign brain tumors.

Benign brain tumors generally develop slowly, have wonderful borders, and do not often spread. Benign tumors can still be dangerous. They can damage and compress components of the brain, causing severe dysfunction. Benign brain tumors positioned in a vital area of the brain can be life-threatening. Very rarely, a benign tumor can emerge as malignant. Examples of generally benign tumors encompass meningioma, vestibular schwannoma, and pituitary adenoma.

Malignant brain tumors are cancerous. They generally grow swiftly and invade surrounding healthful brain structures. Brain cancer can be life-threatening due to the changes it causes to the essential buildings of the brain. Some examples of malignant tumors that originate in or near the brain consist of olfactory neuroblastoma, chondrosarcoma, and medulloblastoma.

Brain Tumor Locations
Brain tumors can shape in any phase of the brain, but there are certain regions where specific tumors form:

- Meningiomas form in the meninges, the protective lining of the brain.

- Pituitary tumors increase in the pituitary gland.
- Medulloblastoma tumors occur from the cerebellum or brainstem.
- Skull base tumors develop on the underside of the brain, referred to as the skull base.

Other brain tumors are described via the kinds of cells they are made of. For instance, gliomas are composed of glial cells.

CHAPTER 2

TYPES OF BRAIN CANCER

There are extra than a hundred and twenty distinct varieties of brain tumors, lesions, and cysts, which can be differentiated with the aid of using wherein they arise and what sorts of cells they may be made from. Certain kinds of tumors are generally benign (noncancerous), even as others are normally malignant (cancerous). Others may also have a 50/50 threat of being cancerous.

Some of the tumor kinds indexed beneath can also additionally rise up from the bone or different styles of tissues outside the brain and can additionally be known as "cranial base tumors." However, their proximity to the brain probably has an effect on the systems of the brain, that's why they're blanketed on this list.

- Typically Benign Tumors
- Other Benign Brain Lesions and Cysts
- Brain Tumors with Variable Grades (From More Benign to Malignant)
- Brain Cancer Types: Typically Malignant Brain Tumors

Typically Benign Brain Tumors
Meningioma

Meningioma is the maximum not unusual place number one brain tumor, accounting for extra than 30% of all brain tumors. Meningiomas originate withinside the meninges, the outer 3 layers of tissue that cowl and guard the brain simply below the cranium. Women are recognized with meningiomas more frequently than men. About 85% of meningiomas are noncancerous, gradual-developing tumors. Almost all meningiomas are taken into consideration benign, however, a few meningiomas may be chronic and are available in the lower back after remedy.

Pituitary Adenoma

Adenoma, a form of tumor that grows withinside the gland tissues, is the maximum not unusual place form of pituitary tumor. Pituitary adenomas increase from the pituitary gland and have a tendency to develop at a sluggish fee. About 10% of number one brain tumors are recognized as adenomas. They can reason imaginative and prescient endocrinological troubles. Fortunately for sufferers stricken by them, adenomas are benign and treatable with surgical treatment and/or medication.

Craniopharyngioma

These benign tumors develop close to the pituitary gland and might seem like strong tumors or cysts. Craniopharyngiomas regularly press on nerves, blood vessels, or components of the brain across the pituitary gland. Like adenomas, they also can motivate imaginative and prescient endocrinological issues. They commonly have an effect on youngsters and young adults in addition to adults over the age of fifty.

Schwannoma

Acoustic neuromas (vestibular schwannomas) are benign, sluggish-developing tumors of the nerve that connects the ear to the brain. Less than 8% of number one brain tumors are acoustic neuromas. They generally expand in center-elderly adults, develop at the nerve sheath — the protection surrounding the nerve fibers — and frequently reason listening to loss. Schwannomas also can have an effect on the trigeminal nerve. These are known as trigeminal schwannomas, which are many less not unusual places than vestibular schwannomas and might motivate facial aches.

Nasopharyngeal Angiofibroma

Nasopharyngeal angiofibroma, additionally called juvenile nasopharyngeal angiofibroma, is a benign cranial base tumor within the nostril that is normally identified in adolescent boys. It is the maximum not unusual place for benign tumors of the nasopharynx (the distance behind the nostril that connects the nostril with the mouth). It spreads to regions across the nostril, inflicting signs consisting of congestion and nosebleeds.

Choroid Plexus Tumor

Choroid plexus tumors are uncommon tumors that are discovered withinside the choroid plexus — the part of the brain inside its ventricles that produces cerebrospinal fluid. About 90% of those tumors are benign. The maximum often arises in kids under the age of two and may cause hydrocephalus, a buildup of cerebrospinal fluid, as they develop. This can bring about improved stress in the brain and expansion of the cranium. An uncommon malignant form of choroid plexus tumor is choroid plexus carcinoma.

Dysembryoplastic Neuroepithelial Tumor

This is a sort of neuronal-glial brain tumor — it's miles made from a mixture of neurons and helping cells. Dysembryoplastic neuroepithelial tumors are uncommon benign tumors that arise withinside the tissues protecting the brain and spinal wire. Typically observed in kids and teenagers, those tumors can cause seizures. Other neuronal-glial brain tumors encompass gangliogliomas, gangliocytomas, and rosette-forming tumors.

Neurofibroma

Neurofibromas are benign, commonly painless tumors that may develop on nerves everywhere withinside the frame. In a few cases, those smooth, fleshy growths expand withinside the brain, on cranial nerves, or at the spinal twine. Multiple neurofibromas are a symptom of a genetic disease known as neurofibromatosis kind 1 (NF1).

Hemangioblastoma

Hemangioblastomas are benign tumors of the blood vessels which can shape withinside the brain. These tumors can frequently be eliminated via a surgical procedure. On uncommon occasions, they could appear on a couple of web websites and be symptomatic of a hereditary ailment referred to as Von Hippel-Lindau. If this is the case, specific exams and visits with an expert which includes an ophthalmologist or geneticist can be endorsed.

Chondroma

Chondromas are very uncommon benign tumor products of cartilage. They can increase withinside the cartilage discovered withinside the cranium base and the paranasal sinuses, however, they also can have an effect on different frame elements which include the palms and feet. Chondromas generally arise in sufferers for a long time of 10 and 30. While those tumors develop slowly, they'll in the end cause the bone to fracture or develop to an awful lot, developing strain on the brain.

Giant Cell Tumor

Named for extraordinarily big cells, massive molecular tumors are uncommon bone tumors that commonly have an effect on the leg and arm bones. They can also be determined withinside the cranium. Most large molecular tumors are benign and arise in sufferers between 20 and forty years of age.

Osteoma

Osteomas are benign bone tumors (new bone growth) that generally increase at the cranium base and facial bones. In general, those gradual-developing tumors have no signs. However, if huge osteomas develop in certain regions of the brain, they'll cause issues with respiration, imagination, and prescient or listening.

Other Benign Brain Lesions and Cysts
Arachnoid Cyst

Arachnoid cysts are not unusual to place benign brain cysts that arise within the membranes surrounding the brain and are full of cerebrospinal fluid. They are normally gifts considering the fact that delivery, motive no signs, and are regularly left untreated.

Colloid Cyst

This is a benign mass that looks withinside the 1/3 ventricle of the brain. It can block the cerebrospinal fluid pathways, inflicting complications and hydrocephalus, or may be determined absolutely incidentally. It is frequently eliminated with surgical operation, in particular, if it causes hydrocephalus.

Dermoid or Epidermoid Cyst

Dermoid and epidermoid cysts are sluggish-developing hundreds that shape from leftover pores and skin tissue in embryonal improvement. They are handled with surgical operation, and follow-up strategies may be performed adequately if entire extirpation isn't feasible throughout the primary surgical treatment.

Encephalocele

Encephalocele is a sac-like protrusion of the brain and the membranes that cowl it through a gap withinside the cranium. This uncommon beginning disorder happens while the neural tube, wherein the brain and spinal twine shape, fails to shut absolutely in the course of fetal improvement. Encephaloceles can arise withinside the base of the cranium, on the pinnacle or lower back of the cranium, or among the brow and nostril. They can reason deformities withinside the face and skull which are repaired with a surgical operation. Each year, approximately one out of each 10,000 babies born within the United States may have an encephalocele, in keeping with the Centers for Disease Control and Prevention.

Fibrous Dysplasia

Fibrous dysplasia is an extraordinary bone ailment wherein scar-like fibrous tissue develops in preference to the everyday bone. As the bone grows, the fibrous tissue steadily expands, weakening the bone. Fibrous dysplasia generally develops withinside the cranium base and facial bones, thighbone, shinbone, ribs, top arm bone, or pelvis. Fibrous dysplasia can result in aches and damaged or deformed bones. Severe deformity of facial bones can cause a lack of imagination and prescient or listening. In uncommon cases, an affected bone vicinity can also additionally end up cancerous.

Rathke's Cleft Cyst

Rathke's cleft cysts are benign fluid-crammed growths that slowly expand withinside the area among the back and front regions of the pituitary gland. Most of Rathke's cleft cysts are discovered in adults, even though they shape all through fetal improvement.

Petrous Apex Lesion

Petrous apex lesions are abnormalities that arise withinside the tip of the bone withinside the cranium subsequent to the center ear. The maximum not unusual place sort of petrous apex lesion is a benign LDL cholesterol granuloma, which is a cyst. Other petrous apex lesions consist of acoustic neuromas and cranial base tumors. Most petrous apex lesions are benign. However, sufferers with different sorts of cancers can also additionally broaden metastatic petrous apex lesions.

Brain Tumors with Variable Grades (From More Benign to Malignant)

Glioma

Glioma is a not unusual place kind of tumor originating withinside the brain, however, it could on occasion be discovered withinside the spinal twine. About 33% of all brain tumors are gliomas. These tumors get up from the glial cells that surround and assist neurons. There are numerous styles of glial cells, and for this reason, there are numerous varieties of gliomas, along with:

Astrocytomas

A not unusual place shape is a pilocytic astrocytoma, a benign brain tumor bobbing up from the assisting brain cells and generally observed in teens or kids. It may be handled with the surgical procedure if the whole tumor may be eliminated.

Oligodendrogliomas

Glioblastomas, an especially competitive kind of tumour. The know-how of gliomas has been evolving over the years. Depending on the kind of cells which might be forming the glioma and their genetic mutations, the tumors may be greater or much less competitive. A genetic observation of the tumor is frequently carried out to better apprehend how it could behave. For example, diffuse midline gliomas or hemispheric gliomas are newly defined kinds of gliomas that have precise mutations related to an extra-competitive nature.

Ependymal Tumors

Ependymal tumors stand up from the liner of the ventricles or the valuable canal of the spinal twine. They are uncommon and might seem at any part of the brain or spinal twine. There are one-of-a-kind sorts, along with:

- Subependymoma
- Myxopapillary ependymoma
- Ependymoma: Similar to gliomas, ependymomas also can have particular

genetic mutations. Their conduct can be exclusive relying on which they're positioned withinside the fearful device.

Hemangiopericytoma

Hemangiopericytomas are uncommon cranial base tumors that contain blood vessels. While maximum hemangiopericytomas are observed in smooth tissues of the legs, pelvic place, head, and neck, a few can also additionally arise withinside the nasal hollow space and paranasal sinuses. These tumors can be benign or malignant.

Germ Cell Tumors

During the everyday improvement of an embryo and fetus, germ cells generally turn out to be eggs (withinside the female) or sperm (withinside the male). However, if germ cells tour the brain through mistake, they could grow to be tumors. Germ molecular tumors may be benign or malignant. Some varieties of germ molecular tumors consist of germinomas, embryonal carcinomas, Yolk sac tumors, and teratomas. They are frequently identified throughout puberty and have a tendency to have an effect on boys more than girls.

Pineal Tumors

Pineal tumors are tumors that seem withinside the place inside the pineal gland. They are deep withinside the brain and may cause hydrocephalus by blocking off the cerebrospinal fluid pathways. There are extraordinary varieties of pineal tumors with wonderful behaviors, together with pineocytomas, pineal parenchymal tumors of intermediate differentiation, and pineoblastoma. Other tumors this sort as gliomas, teratomas, and germ molecular tumors can seem withinside the pineal place. A blood check or a lumbar puncture can be endorsed to search for markers that could assist in the analysis of a pineal tumor. In different instances, a surgical procedure for biopsy is endorsed.

Brain Cancer Types: Typically Malignant Brain Tumors
Chordoma

Chordomas are an extraordinary shape of bone most cancers are commonly determined withinside the base of the cranium or the decrease again. Less than 1% of all number one brain tumors are recognized as chordomas. This kind of tumor can invade adjoining bones and place a strain on nearby nerve tissue. Although this tumor is gradual-developing and appears reputedly benign, it behaves extra like a malignant tumor due to its tendency to return back again and unfold to different regions. Chordomas, at the same time as usually competitive, have a quite variable and unpredictable progression.

Chondrosarcoma

Chondrosarcoma is a malignant bone most cancers that especially impacts cartilage. Chondrosarcoma typically develops in sufferers between the age of fifty and 70. The tumor can start in cells within the thigh bone, arm, pelvis, knee, and spine. It may additionally begin within the facial bones or cranium base. Some of those cancers may be competitive.

Medulloblastoma

Medulloblastoma is the maximum not unusual place for malignant brain tumors in kids. It normally impacts kids among a long time five and 9 and is uncommon in humans over 30. It arises withinside the cerebellum, part of the brain positioned at the bottom of the cranium. There are one-of-a-kind varieties of medulloblastoma, and their aggressivity may also extrude relying on precise mutations of the tumor cells.

Olfactory Neuroblastoma

Olfactory neuroblastoma, additionally referred to as esthesioneuroblastoma, is a completely uncommon malignant tumor that develops within the nostril. This tumor possibly begins withinside the olfactory nerve, which transmits impulses associated with odor from the nostril to the brain. Patients with olfactory neuroblastomas might also additionally revel in common nosebleeds, lose their experience of odor, and feature problem respiration thru their nostrils.

Lymphoma

Lymphoma is a kind of tumor that paperwork in a part of the frame's immune machine, the lymphatic device. Lymphomas can unfold from different frame elements to the brain or shape withinside the brain (number one crucial anxious machine lymphomas). Surgery can be endorsed to verify the tumor kind with a biopsy, however, number one CNS lymphomas are extra frequently dealt with chemotherapy and radiation.

Gliosarcoma

These tumors are uncommon sorts of glioma combined with different supportive tissues. Gliosarcomas can unfold to different regions and are normally competitive and immune to therapy.

Rhabdomyosarcoma

Rhabdomyosarcoma is an unprecedented shape of tender tissue most cancers form the muscle. While it may arise in lots of locations within the frame, along with the hands and legs, it's far more frequently located withinside the head and neck and the cranium base. Children are much more likely to increase rhabdomyosarcomas. This can gift with issues within the eyes or face. Certain inherited conditions, which include neurofibromatosis kind 1 (NF1), grow the hazard of this ailment.

Paranasal Sinus Cancer

Cancer of the paranasal sinuses bureaucracy withinside the tissues lining the hole areas withinside the bones across the nostril. This malignant cranium base tumor is more often than not observed withinside the maxillary sinuses (withinside the cheekbones below the eyes) and the ethmoid sinuses (besides the top nostril). There are extraordinary kinds of cancers withinside the paranasal sinuses and remedy may also consist of a mixture of surgical treatment, radiation, and chemotherapy.

Atypical Teratoid/Rhabdoid Tumor (AT/RT)

AT/RT is an extraordinary sort of embryonal tumor of the important worried machine. It commonly influences kids 6 and younger, it's miles fast-developing, and the survival price is low despite competitive surgical procedures, radiation, and chemotherapy.

CHAPTER 3

CAUSES OF BRAIN CANCER

Researchers know brain tumors boost when positive genes on the chromosomes of a cell phone are broken and no longer characteristic properly, but they aren't positive why this happens. The DNA in your chromosomes tells cells throughout your physique what to do — it tells them when to grow, when to divide or multiply and/or when to die.

The causes of brain cancer are still largely unknown. Although some genetic stipulations and environmental elements can also contribute to the improvement of Brain cancer, the hazard elements are an awful lot much less defined for brain cancer than for other cancers in the body. Also, the chance of developing essential brain cancers is very low. The American Cancer

Society estimates the hazard over a lifetime is less than 1 percent.

It's necessary to take note that the brain most cancers chance factor solely impacts the likelihood of creating brain cancer over a lifetime. For example, if you've obtained radiation remedy to deal with any other cancer, or if you've labored in an industry where you treated doubtlessly cancerous chemicals, you may also want to discuss with your doctor what it is capable of for your character's chance of creating Brain cancer.

There is no definitive purpose for most important brain tumors or brain cancer. Secondary brain tumors, or brain metastases, are cancers that originate in other components of the physique and unfold to the brain. They are some distance extra frequent than predominant brain tumors. The risk aspect for secondary Brain cancers depends on the place cancer originated. The most common principal cancers that spread to the brain encompass breast, lung, kidney, colorectal, and melanoma.

When brain cell DNA changes, it gives your brain cells new instructions. Your physique develops unusual brain cells that develop and multiply faster than regular and sometimes stay longer than normal. When that happens, the ever-growing crowd of bizarre cells takes over space in your brain.

In some cases, a man or woman may additionally be born with adjustments in one or greater of these genes. Environmental factors, such as exposure to massive quantities of radiation from X-rays or preceding cancer treatment, may additionally then lead to further damage.

In different cases, environmental injury to the genes can also be the sole cause.

There are a few rare, inherited (passed down from father or mother to child) genetic syndromes that are related to brain tumors, including:

- Neurofibromatosis kind 1 (NF1 gene).
- Neurofibromatosis kind two (NF2 gene).
- Turcot syndrome (APC gene).
- Gorlin syndrome (PTCH gene).
- Tuberous sclerosis complex (TSC1 and TSC2 genes).
- Li-Fraumeni syndrome (TP53 gene).

Only about 5% to 10% of human beings with brain tumors have a family record of a brain tumor.

CHAPTER 4

RISK FACTORS OF BRAIN CANCER

Here, a chance issue is something that increases a person's chance of creating a brain tumor. Although risk factors regularly affect the improvement of a brain tumor, most no longer immediately cause a brain tumor. Some humans with several risk factors never boost a brain tumor, whilst others with no recognized risk elements do. Knowing your hazard factors and speaking about them with your doctor may additionally assist you to make more knowledgeable decisions. But, at this time, there are no acknowledged ways to prevent a brain tumor through way of life changes.

Most of the time, the motive of a brain tumor is unknown, however, the following elements may additionally elevate a person's threat of growing a brain tumor:

Age

Brain tumors are more common in youth and older adults, even though humans of any age can strengthen a brain tumor.

Gender

In general, men are more likely than females to increase brain tumors. However, some precise sorts of brain tumors, such as meningioma, are more frequent in women.

Home And Work Exposures

Exposure to solvents, pesticides, oil products, rubber, or vinyl chloride may also enlarge the danger of growing a brain tumor. However, there is now no scientific proof that supports this viable link.

Family History

About 5% of brain tumors may be linked to hereditary genetic factors or conditions, which include Li-Fraumeni syndrome, neurofibromatosis, nevoid basal phone carcinoma syndrome, tuberous sclerosis, Turcot syndrome, and von Hippel-Lindau disease. Scientists have additionally observed "clusters" of brain tumors inside some households except a link to these recognized hereditary conditions. Studies are underway to attempt to discover a motive for these clusters.

Exposure To Infections, Viruses, And Allergens

Infection with the Epstein-Barr virus (EBV) will increase the chance of CNS lymphoma. EBV is typically recognized as the virus that motivates mononucleosis or "mono." In other research, high tiers of a frequent virus called cytomegalovirus (CMV) have been discovered in brain tumor tissue. The means of this finding is being researched. Several sorts of other viruses have been proven to cause brain tumors in research on animals. More information is needed to discover if exposure to infections, different viruses, or allergens enlarge the danger of a brain tumor in people. Of note, research has proven that sufferers with a history of hypersensitive reactions or skin conditions have a lower danger of glioma.

Electromagnetic Fields

Most studies evaluating the function of electromagnetic fields, such as electricity from electricity traces or mobile phone smartphone use, exhibit no link to a multiplied threat of developing a brain tumor in adults. Because of conflicting statistics regarding chance in children, the World Health Organization (WHO) recommends limiting cell telephone use and promoting the use of a hands-free headset for each adult and children.

Race And Ethnicity

In the United States, white human beings are more probable to boost gliomas but less probable to enhance meningioma than Black people. Also, humans from northern Europe are more than twice as likely to increase brain tumors as people in Japan.

Ionizing Radiation

Previous treatment of the brain or head with ionizing radiation, including x-rays, is a risk issue for a brain tumor.

Head Injury And Seizures

Serious head trauma has long been studied for its relationship to brain tumors. Some research has shown a hyperlink between head trauma and meningioma however no longer between head trauma and glioma. A record of seizures has also been linked with brain tumors, however, due to the fact a brain tumor can cause seizures, it is not known if seizures make the risk of brain tumors bigger, if seizures show up due to the fact of the tumor, or if anti-seizure remedy will increase the risk.

N-nitroso Compounds

Some studies of weight loss programs and vitamin supplementation appear to point out that dietary N-nitroso compounds might also raise the risk of both childhood and personal brain tumors. Dietary N-nitroso compounds are shaped in the body from nitrites or nitrates located in some cured meats, cigarette smoke, and cosmetics. However, extra lookup is essential before a definitive hyperlink can be established.

CHAPTER 5

SYMPTOMS OF BRAIN CANCER

People with a brain tumor would possibly also time out the following signs and signs and symptoms or signs. A symptom is something that solely the character experiencing it can discover and describe, such as fatigue, nausea, or pain. A signal is something that other people can pick out and measure, such as a fever, rash, or an improved pulse. Together, signs and symptoms and symptoms and symptoms can assist describe a clinical problem. Sometimes, human beings with brain tumors do not have any of the signs and signs and symptoms described below. Or, the purpose of a symptom or sign may additionally be a scientific circumstance that is no longer a brain tumor.

Who Do Brain Tumors Affect?

Brain tumors have an effect on early life and adults and can reinforce at any age. They're barely more regularly occurring in human beings assigned male at the transport (AMAB) than human beings assigned lady at the start (AFAB).

Meningioma, which is usually benign, is the only form of brain tumor that's greater common in human beings AFAB.

The most serious type of brain tumor, glioblastoma, is turning into a larger frequent amongst people who are as the everyday populace ages.

Symptoms of a brain tumor can be widespread or specific. A vast symptom is precipitated with the aid of the stress of the tumor on the brain or spinal cord. Specific symptoms are brought on when a unique phase of the brain is no longer working nicely due to the fact of the tumor. Many human beings with a brain tumor, were diagnosed when they went to the physician after experiencing a problem, such as a headache or exclusive changes.

General Signs And Symptoms Include:

1. **Headaches**, which may moreover be excessive and irritate with the undertaking or in the early morning

2. **Seizures.** People can also additionally journey one of the form varieties of seizures. Certain tablets can assist, end or manipulate them. Motor seizures, additionally known as convulsions, are surprising involuntary movements of a person's muscles. The one-of-a-kind kinds of seizures and what they show up like are listed below:

Myoclonic

- Single or a couple of muscle twitches, jerks, spasms

- Tonic-Clonic (Grand Mal)

- Loss of recognition and physique tone followed through the usage of twitching and enjoyable muscle organizations that are referred to as contractions

- Loss of management of body functions, such as loss of bladder control

- Maybe a quick 30-second length of no breathing and a person's pores and pores and skin can additionally flip a coloration of blue, purple, gray, white, or green

- After this type of seizure, a man or lady may additionally moreover be sleepy and experience a headache, confusion, weakness, numbness, and sore muscles

Sensory

- Change in sensation, vision, smell, and/or listening to barring dropping consciousness

Complex Partial

- May reason a loss of consciousness or a partial or complete loss of consciousness

- May be associated with repetitive, unintentional movements, such as twitching

3. Personality or reminiscence changes

4. Nausea or vomiting

5. Fatigue

6. Drowsiness

7. Sleep problems

8. Memory problems

9. Changes in the potential to stroll or function in daily activities

Symptoms that may additionally be unique to the place of the tumor include:

- Pressure or headache close to the tumor.

- Loss of steadiness and challenge with quality motor abilities is linked with a tumor in the cerebellum.

- Changes in judgment, consisting of loss of initiative, sluggishness, and muscle weak factor or paralysis associated with a tumor in the frontal lobe of the cerebrum.

- Partial or total loss of vision is precipitated with the aid of the ability of a tumor in the occipital lobe or temporal lobe of the cerebrum.

- Changes in speech, hearing, memory, or emotional state, such as aggressiveness and issues grasping or retrieving phrases can improve from a tumor in the frontal and temporal lobe of the cerebrum.

- Altered perception of contact or pressure, arm or leg susceptible spot on 1 facet of the body, or confusion with left and applicable aspects of the physique are linked to a tumor in the frontal or parietal lobe of the cerebrum.

- The inability to appear upward can be precipitated via the capability of a pineal gland tumor.

- Lactation, which is the secretion of breast milk, and altered menstrual periods, as nicely as amplified in arms and toes in the course of adulthood, are linked with a pituitary tumor.

- Difficulty swallowing, facial weak factor or numbness, or double ingenious and prescient is a symptom of a tumor in the brain stem.

- Vision changes, which encompass loss of a section of the imaginative and prescient or double vision can be from a tumor in the temporal lobe, occipital lobe, or brain stem.

If you are worried about any modifications you experience, please discuss them with your doctor. Your clinical physician will ask how long and how often you've been experiencing the symptom(s), in addition to other questions. This is to help determine the cause of the problem, called a diagnosis.

If a brain tumor is diagnosed, relieving signs and symptoms stays a crucial phase of your care and treatment. This may additionally be referred to as "palliative care" or "supportive care." It regularly commenced quickly after prognosis and persevered in the direction of treatment. Be sure to speak with your health care team about the signs and symptoms and symptoms you experience, inclusive of any new signs or a change in symptoms.

CHAPTER 6

PREVENTION OF BRAIN CANCER

Researchers say that most instances of brain cancer don't have a clear cause, but exposure to radiation and a household history of brain tumors may additionally enlarge your risk. Typically, brain cancer takes place when tumors develop inside your brain or near it. Although most cancers might also originate in your brain, it's additionally viable for most cancers to spread to your brain from other areas of your body.

Experts agree that cancerous tumors commonly enhance after your mobile DNA is altered, but, unfortunately, researchers are still attempting to figure out what lifestyle elements may make contributions to brain cancer. If you're concerned about cancer, dwelling on a wholesome lifestyle and getting wellness assessments might also help you guard your health.

Be Aware Of Your Risk.

Doctors do not now recognize what motives brain cancer in most cases, but certain factors can make your risk bigger. Knowing these elements can assist you to discover your threat and viable symptoms, and getting ordinary checkups.

The principal threat elements for brain cancers include age, publicity to radiation, a family history of brain tumors, and currently having most cancers that should metastasize (spread) to your brain from some other region of your body.

The brain, like the liver and lungs, has a lot of blood vessels. If a "seed" of cancer travels from somewhere else in the body, the possibility of it settling in these areas with many blood vessels is higher. This is why having cancer elsewhere in your body puts you at extended risk.

Recognize Your Threat Increases With Age.

Any person, from youth to the elderly, can strengthen brain cancer; however, your hazard for the sickness increases the older you get. Recognizing this and being conscious of your body may assist you to seek a clinical opinion if you note any symptoms of brain cancer.

Some brain tumors and cancer, such as brainstem gliomas and astrocytomas, are nearly exclusively present in children.

Ask About Your Family's Scientific History.
Keep an exact report of your family's scientific history, inclusive of instances of cancer and tumors. If you have a family history of brain tumors or positive genetic syndromes that extend the risk for brain cancer, you are at a higher hazard of growing most cancers of the brain or surrounding areas. Understanding your family's scientific records of brain cancer can pick out workable signs and cure options.

- It's always smart to hold a non-public document of your family's clinical history and to have one at your doctor's office.

- Only 5 – 10% of all cancers are hereditary.
- A household record of Li-Fraumeni syndrome, neurofibromatosis, tuberous sclerosis, and Turcot syndrome might also make you more susceptible to brain cancer.

The reasons for brain cancer are no longer nicely understood, and as such, there are no guaranteed methods to stop the disease. However, there are some matters that you can do to lower your chance of developing brain cancer:

Limit Publicity To Radiation.
Different kinds of radiation can enlarge your hazard of growing brain cancer. Limiting your radiation exposure may also assist you to prevent the development of the disease.

Ionizing radiation, which is currently in some radiation treatment options for cancer or atomic bombs, will increase your risk of brain cancer. You may additionally now not be in a position to

limit your exposure to ionizing radiation if you are present process therapy for any other cancer. The possibility of being uncovered thru an atomic bomb or nuclear meltdown is low.
Ultraviolet radiation, which the solar emits, can additionally make your risk for brain cancer bigger. Wearing sunscreen and a head cover and limiting sun exposure may also limit your risk.

Understand What Types Of Radiation Do Now Not Cause Brain Cancer.
People are regularly exposed to greater common forms of radiation consisting of electromagnetic fields or radiofrequency radiation. Although some people consider that these types of radiation cause brain cancer, there is no proof linking them to brain tumors.

- Studies have now not linked radiation from electricity lines, cellphone phones, smartphones, or microwaves to brain cancer.

- Stay abreast of research on radiation exposure, which may additionally assist identify your hazard factors.

Change Your Consuming And Nutritional Habits.

There is some evidence that nutritional habits for the duration of fetal development, childhood, and adulthood may additionally minimize your risk of creating brain cancer. Eating masses of fruits and greens and decreasing cholesterol may also assist you to stop brain cancer.

If your mom ate fruits and greens all through her pregnancy and/or gave them to you as a part of your weight loss program throughout childhood, you can also be at a lower danger of creating brain cancer.

Continuing to devour a food plan rich in distinctive fruits and vegetables may additionally maintain your danger for brain cancer lower.

Lowering your LDL cholesterol and limiting how many fatty meals you consume may additionally reduce your hazard for brain cancer.

Exercise Regularly.
Aim to exercise most days of the week. Doing a cardiovascular workout can assist you to continue to be wholesome and may minimize your danger of creating brain cancer.

You can do any type of cardio education to keep your health. Beyond walking, reflect on the consideration of running, swimming, rowing, or biking.

Wear Defensive Headgear.
If you participate in things that put you at risk of head injury, such as contact sports, make certain to put on a helmet or different terrific headgear to shield your head.

Eat A Wholesome Diet.
A food regimen wealthy in fruits, vegetables, total grains, and lean proteins can assist standard fitness and might also lower your threat of creating cancer.

Avoid Smoking And Immoderate Alcohol Consumption.

Both smoking and heavy alcohol consumption have been linked to an improved threat of a variety of types of cancer, such as brain cancer. If you do smoke or drink, strive to give up or limit your use.

It's necessary to preserve the idea that whilst these techniques may lower your threat of developing brain cancer, they are no longer foolproof. Regular check-ups with a healthcare professional can assist with the early detection and treatment of brain cancer.

CHAPTER 7

DIAGNOSIS OF BRAIN CANCER

If your healthcare company thinks you might have a brain tumor, you'll need a number of exams and procedures to be sure. These would possibly include:

A Neurological Exam.
A neurological examination tests exclusive parts of your brain to see how they're working. This exam may additionally include checking your vision, hearing, balance, coordination, power, and reflexes. If you have bothered in one or more areas, this is a clue for your healthcare provider. A neurological examination doesn't observe a brain tumor. But it helps your company apprehend what part of your brain might be having a problem.

Head CT Scan.

A computed tomography scan, additionally known as a CT scan, makes use of X-rays to make pictures. It's broadly available, and effects come again quickly. So CT may be the first imaging check that truly is executed if you have complications or different signs and symptoms that have many viable causes. A CT scan can become aware of troubles in and around your brain. The effects provide your fitness care provider clues to figure out what checks to do next. If your provider thinks your CT scan indicates a brain tumor, you may need a brain MRI.

Brain MRI.

Magnetic resonance imaging, also known as MRI, uses strong magnets to create pix of the internal organs of the body. MRI is regularly used to realize brain tumors due to the fact it suggests the brain extra in reality than other imaging tests.

Often a dye is injected into a vein in the arm before an MRI. The dye makes clearer pictures.

This makes it less difficult to see smaller tumors. It can assist your fitness care team see the distinction between a brain tumor and healthy brain tissue.

Sometimes you want a distinctive kind of MRI to create more detailed pictures. One instance is practical MRI. This one-of-a-kind MRI shows which components of the brain manage to speak, move, and different necessary tasks. This helps your fitness care provider graph surgical procedures and different treatments.

Magnetic Resonance Spectroscopy.
This is another exclusive MRI test. This uses MRI to measure tiers of certain chemicals in the tumor cells. Having too much or too little of the chemicals may tell your fitness care crew about the form of brain tumor you have.

Magnetic resonance perfusion is another exceptional kind of MRI. This test uses MRI to measure the amount of blood in different parts of the brain tumor. The parts of the tumor that have a greater quantity of blood may also be the most active parts of the tumor. Your healthcare team makes use of these statistics to design your treatment.

PET Scan Of The Brain.

A positron emission tomography scan, additionally called a PET scan, can become aware of some brain tumors. A PET scan makes use of a radioactive tracer it is injected into a vein. The tracer travels via the blood and attaches to brain tumor cells. The tracer makes the tumor cells stand out in the photos taken using the PET machine. Cells that are dividing and multiplying shortly will take up greater of the tracer.

A PET scan may be most helpful for detecting brain tumors that are growing quickly. Examples include glioblastomas and some oligodendrogliomas. Brain tumors that grow slowly might now not be detected on a PET scan. Brain tumors that don't seem to be cancerous tend to develop more slowly, so PET scans are less beneficial for benign brain tumors. Not everybody with a brain tumor wants a PET scan. Ask your healthcare company whether or not you want a PET scan.

Collecting A Sample Of Tissue.
A brain biopsy is a system to take away a pattern of brain tumor tissue for checking out in a lab. Often a physician gets the pattern at some stage in surgery to get rid of the brain tumor.

If surgical treatment isn't always possible, a pattern may be removed with a needle. Removing a pattern of brain tumor tissue with a needle is done with a technique referred to as stereotactic needle biopsy.

During this procedure, a small gap is drilled into the skull. A thin needle is inserted through the hole. The needle is used to take a tissue sample. Imaging assessments such as CT and MRI are used to format the direction of the needle. You might not experience whatever at some point during the biopsy due to the fact a remedy is used to numb the area. Often you also obtain medicine that places you in a sleep-like state so you are no longer aware.

You may have a needle biopsy alternatively than surgical treatment if your healthcare crew is concerned that an operation might harm an essential section of your brain. A needle might be wished to do away with tissue from a brain tumor if the tumor is in a spot that's challenging to attain with surgery.

Brain biopsy has a risk of complications. Risks encompass bleeding in the brain and harm to the brain tissue.

Testing The Tissue Sample In The Lab. The biopsy sample is despatched to a lab for testing. Tests can see whether or not the cells are cancerous or no longer cancerous. The way the cells appear beneath a microscope can inform your fitness care crew how rapidly the cells are growing. This is known as the brain tumor's grade. Other exams can find out what DNA

modifications are currently in the cells. This
helps your fitness care team create your cure
plan.

CHAPTER 8

TREATMENT FOR BRAIN CANCER

Treatment for a brain tumor relies upon whether or not the tumor is a brain most cancers or if it is now no longer cancerous, additionally referred to as a benign brain tumor. Treatment alternatives additionally rely on the sort, size, grade, and area of the brain tumor. Options would possibly encompass surgical procedures, radiation remedies, radiosurgery, chemotherapy, and centered remedies. When thinking about your remedy alternatives, your fitness care group additionally considers your normal fitness and your preferences.

Treatment may not be wanted properly away. You may not want to remedy properly in case your brain tumor is small, is not cancerous, and would not motivate symptoms. Small, benign brain tumors won't develop or would possibly develop so slowly that they might not ever reason problems. You would possibly have brain MRI scans in some instances a year to test for brain tumor growth. If the brain tumor grows extra quicker than anticipated or in case you expand symptoms, you would possibly want a remedy.

Surgery

The purpose of surgical treatment for a brain tumor is to put off all the tumor cells. The tumor can not usually be eliminated completely. When it is possible, the medical professional works to take away as much of the brain tumor as may be performed safely. Brain tumor elimination surgical procedures may be used to deal with brain cancers and benign brain tumors.

Some brain tumors are small and smooth to split from surrounding brain tissue. This makes it probable that the tumor could be eliminated completely. Other brain tumors can not be separated from surrounding tissue. Sometimes a brain tumor is close to a crucial part of the brain.

Surgery is probably unstable in this situation. The doctor may take out a great deal of the tumor as is safe. Removing all parts of a brain tumor is from time to time known as a subtotal resection.

Removal of a part of your brain tumor may also assist lessen your symptoms.

There are many methods of doing brain tumor elimination surgical treatment. Which alternative is high-quality for you relies upon your situation. Examples of kinds of brain tumor surgical treatment consist of:

Removing a part of the cranium to get to the brain tumor. A brain surgical procedure that includes casting off a part of the cranium is referred to as craniotomy. It's the manner maximum brain tumor elimination operations are finished. Craniotomy is used for treating cancerous brain tumors and benign brain tumors.

The health care professional makes a reduction to your scalp. The pores and skin and muscular tissues are moved out of the manner. Then the health care professional makes use of a drill to reduce a segment of the cranium bone. The bone is eliminated to get admission to the brain. If the tumor is deep withinside the brain, a device is probably used to softly keep healthful brain tissue out of the manner. The brain tumor is reduced with unique equipment. Sometimes lasers are used to ruin the tumor.

During the surgical procedure, you obtain the medicinal drug to numb the place so that you might not experience anything. You're additionally given a remedy that places you in a sleep-like kingdom at some point of surgical treatment. Sometimes you're awake for the duration of a brain surgical operation. This is referred to as a wide-conscious brain surgical procedure. When you are awake, the healthcare professional would possibly ask questions and display the hobby for your brain as you respond.

This facilitates a decrease in the danger of injuring critical components of the brain.

When the tumor elimination surgical operation is finished, the part of the cranium bone is positioned and returned to place.

Using a long, skinny tube to get to the brain tumor. Endoscopic brain surgical operation includes placing a long, skinny tube into the brain. The tube is referred to as an endoscope. The tube has a chain of lenses or a tiny digital digicam that transmits photographs to the general practitioner. Special equipment is positioned thru the tube to take away the tumor.

Endoscopic brain surgical procedure is frequently used to deal with pituitary tumors. These tumors develop simply at the back of the nasal cavity. The long, skinny tube is placed thru the nostril and sinuses and into the brain.

Sometimes endoscopic brain surgical treatment is used to take away brain tumors in different elements of the brain. The healthcare provider may use a drill to make a hollow withinside the cranium. The long, skinny tube is cautiously placed via the brain tissue. The tube is maintained till it reaches the brain tumor.

Surgery to do away with a brain tumor has a chance of aspect outcomes and complications. These can encompass infection, bleeding, blood clots, and damage to the brain tissue. Other dangers may also depend upon the part of the brain in which the tumor is located. For instance, a surgical procedure on a tumor close to nerves that hook up with the eyes would possibly have a danger of imaginative and prescient loss. Surgery to get rid of a tumor on a nerve that controls listening to and listening to reason.

Radiation Remedy
Radiation remedy for brain tumors makes use of effective power beams to kill tumor cells. Electricity can come from X-rays, protons, and different sources. Radiation remedy for brain tumors typically comes from a system out of

doors. This is known as outside beam radiation. Rarely, the radiation may be positioned in the frame. This is referred to as brachytherapy.

Radiation remedies may be used to deal with brain cancers and benign brain tumors.

External beam radiation remedy is commonly achieved in quick day-by-day remedies. An ordinary remedy plan would possibly contain having radiation remedies 5 days every week for two to six weeks.

External beam radiation can be sensed simply at the region of your brain in which the tumor is located, or it could be implemented in your whole brain. Most human beings with a brain tumor can have radiation aimed toward the region across the tumor. If there are numerous tumors, the complete brain may want radiation remedy. When the brain is treated, it is referred to as whole-brain radiation. Whole-brain radiation is most customarily used to deal with most cancers that spread to the brain from some other part of the frame and bureaucracy more than one tumor withinside the brain.

Traditionally, radiation remedy makes use of X-rays, however, a more modern shape of this remedy makes use of strength from protons. The proton beams may be extra cautiously centered to most effectively harm the tumor cells. They can be much less probable to harm close healthful tissue. Proton remedy can be useful for treating brain tumors in kids. It additionally may also assist in treating tumors which can be very near essential components of the brain. Proton remedy is not as extensively to be had as conventional X-ray radiation remedy.

Side consequences of radiation remedy for brain tumors rely upon the sort and dose of radiation you get hold of. Common aspect results that show up at some point of remedy or proper after it are fatigue, headaches, reminiscence loss, scalp inflammation, and hair loss. Sometimes radiation remedy facet results display up a few years later. These past-due facet outcomes would possibly consist of reminiscence and questioning problems.

Radiosurgery

Stereotactic radiosurgery for brain tumors is an excessive shape of radiation remedy. It targets beams of radiation from many angles on the brain tumor. Each beam is not very effective. But the factor wherein the beams meet receives a totally big dose of radiation that kills the tumor cells.

Radiosurgery may be used to deal with brain cancers and benign brain tumors.

There are exceptional styles of era utilized in radiosurgery to supply radiation to deal with brain tumors. Some examples consist of:

- Linear accelerator radiosurgery. Linear accelerator machines are also referred to as LINAC machines. LINAC machines are acknowledged with the aid of using their emblem names, which include

CyberKnife, TrueBeam, and others. LINAC gadget objectives cautiously formed beams of power one after the other from numerous exclusive angles. The beams are made from X-rays.

- Gamma Knife radiosurgery. A Gamma Knife device goals many small beams of radiation at an equal time. The beams are made from gamma rays.
- Proton radiosurgery. Proton radiosurgery makes use of beams of protons. This is the most modern form of radiosurgery. It's turning into an extra not unusual place however isn't always to be had in any respect hospitals.
- Radiosurgery is usually accomplished in a single remedy or some remedies. You can cross domestic after remedy and do not want to live in a hospital.

Side results of radiosurgery consist of feeling very worn-out and pores and skin adjustments for your scalp. The pores and skin in your head can also additionally sense dry, itchy, and sensitive. You may have blisters in the pores and skin or hair loss. Sometimes the hair loss is permanent.

Chemotherapy

Chemotherapy for brain tumors makes use of robust drugs to kill tumor cells. Chemotherapy drugs may be taken in tablet shape or injected right into a vein. Sometimes the chemotherapy remedy is located withinside the brain tissue all through surgical operation.

Chemotherapy may be used to deal with brain cancers and benign brain tumors. Sometimes it is performed at an equal time as a radiation remedy.

Chemotherapy aspect consequences rely upon the sort and dose of medicine you get hold of. Chemotherapy can cause nausea, vomiting, and hair loss.

Targeted Remedy

Targeted remedy for brain tumors makes use of drugs that assault unique chemical substances in the tumor cells. By blocking off those chemical compounds, focused remedies can motivate tumor cells to die.

Targeted remedy drugs are to be had for sure sorts of brain cancers and benign brain tumors. Your brain tumor cells can be examined to see whether or not a focused remedy is probably that will help you.

Recovering After Remedy
After the remedy, you may want to assist to regain features withinside the part of your brain that had the tumor. You may want to assist with moving, speaking, seeing, and questioning. Based on your particular needs, your fitness care issuer would possibly suggest:

- Physical remedy that will help you regain misplaced motor capabilities or muscle strength.

- Occupational remedy that will help you get again into your ordinary day-by-day activities, along with work.
- Speech remedy to assist if talking is difficult.
- Tutoring for school-age kids to assist them to deal with modifications of their reminiscence and questioning.

CHAPTER 9

COMPLICATIONS OF BRAIN CANCER TREATMENTS

The aspect outcomes of most cancer remedies can range relying upon the kind of remedy received, the place and length of the tumor, and the person's patient's fitness and clinical history. Here are a number of the maximum, not unusual place aspect consequences related to brain most cancers treatments:

Surgery

Surgery to do away with a brain tumor can motivate several aspects of outcomes, along with headache, swelling, infection, bleeding, and adjustments in imaginative and prescient or speech. The region of the tumor and the quantity of the surgical procedure also can cause different aspects of results, consisting of weak points or paralysis in one facet of the body, the problem with stability or coordination, or seizures.

Radiation Remedy

Radiation remedies can cause fatigue, hair loss, pores and skin inflammation or discoloration, headaches, and nausea. Long-time period aspect results may also consist of cognitive modifications and an expanded danger of growing different styles of most cancers.

Chemotherapy

Chemotherapy can motivate various aspects of consequences, consisting of nausea, vomiting, hair loss, fatigue, and a better hazard of infection. Long-time period aspect consequences might also additionally encompass harm to the coronary heart, lungs, or kidneys, and a multiplied danger of growing different forms of most cancers.

Targeted Remedy

Targeted remedy capsules can cause pores and skin rashes, diarrhea, fatigue, and an elevated danger of infection. Some focused remedy capsules also can motivate extra extreme facet results, together with coronary heart troubles or liver harm.

Immunotherapy

Immunotherapy pills can motivate flu-like symptoms, fatigue, pores and skin rash, and a better danger of infection. Some immunotherapy pills also can cause greater severe side effects, including infection of the lungs or liver.

It's crucial to maintain in the brain that now no longer all sufferers will revel in those aspect outcomes and that the aspect results can frequently be controlled with remedies or different treatments. Patients ought to paint carefully with their healthcare group to control any facet results and to expand a plan for post-remedy care and follow-up.

CHAPTER 10

COPING AND SUPPORT

Every remedy for a brain tumor can purposely face results or modifications on your frame and the way you sense. For many reasons, humans do now no longer revel in the identical aspect consequences even if they're given the identical remedy for the identical sort of tumor. This could make it difficult to expect how you'll sense at some stage in remedy.

As you put together to begin remedy, it's far too ordinary to worry about remedy-associated facet results. It may also assist to recognise that your fitness care group will paint to save you and relieve aspect results. This part of the remedy is known as "palliative care" or "supportive care." It is a crucial part of your remedy plan, no matter your age or the level of disease.

Coping With Personality Changes

Depression, anger, confusion, and mood swings are common signs and symptoms for humans with brain tumors. Personality swings are triggered by the tumor, the treatment, or when you sense hopelessness. In all cases, these modifications can be very tough to manage, whether or not they are small or drastic.

Speak with your doctor if you are aware of these sorts of changes. Many emotional shifts can be handled with medication, and you can find help to help you through these tough times.

Coping With Cognitive & Behavioral Changes

A brain tumor and its treatment(s) can cause adjustments in your conduct and capability to think. You may also have a hard time with communication, concentration, memory, and feeling moody. These difficulties can certainly affect your everyday life, and they do not usually go away. This can motivate stress for all of us involved.

Medicine and counseling may also be prescribed to help control cognitive and behavioral changes. Cognitive rehabilitation equipment can assist too.

Coping with Anxiety & Depression
Feeling anxious from the tumor or therapy is very common, but it makes every scene feel more intense. Often, despair is felt with anxiety. Treatments encompass relaxation techniques, antianxiety and/or antidepressant medications, and counseling. Talking about how you sense with anyone knowledgeable in relieving emotional issues can help.

- Symptoms of anxiousness include rapid heartbeat, fear, restlessness, nervousness, and sweaty palms. If you sense anxiety it is vital to discuss it. It's the first step to regaining management in your life.

- Symptoms of melancholy include: feeling irritable, hopeless and unable to concentrate, withdrawn, and moody. Some people want to damage themselves. Depression is serious. It can and must be dealt with on its own.

- Most people say that their mood improves as the signs and facets consequences of a brain tumor or its cure are managed and go away.

Coping With Headaches

Headaches are most frequently prompted by employing edema. Edema is swelling of the brain brought about using the tumor or treatment. Steroids may additionally be prescribed to minimize edema, but steroids can cause their set of issues (difficulty sleeping, sweating, over-eating, agitation, leg weakness). If you take steroids, inform your clinical group if you can't sleep or have other new signs so they can regulate the dose. Avastin, a drug regularly used to treat glioblastomas, is also very useful in decreasing edema.

Some complications are linked to dizziness, nausea, or vomiting. This is frequently linked to the location of the tumor in the brain. The surgical removal of the tumor will regularly relieve these headaches. Post-operative headaches regularly go away after a brief period.

If your complications don't go away or if they return, it should be a sign of recurrent edema or a new tumor. This must be addressed by your cure team.

Coping With Seizures

A seizure is when a bizarre burst of electrical undertaking in the brain motives an attack. It can motivate muscle contractions, staring, or a loss of consciousness. Some humans solely trip one seizure, while others go through many. They are extra common with slow-growing tumors such as low-grade gliomas but can manifest with most types of tumors.

A patient may be put on an antiepileptic (AED) or antiseizure drug to prevent future seizures. The kind and amount of AED medicinal drugs are based totally on your signs and how nicely you react to it. Also, some AEDs need to no longer be used with chemotherapy.

Patients with seizures that affect awareness (complex partial seizures and generalized seizures) typically cannot drive for a duration of time. The genuine duration varies with the laws of every state.

Patients who have many seizures can preserve a journal to keep track. Write down when they happen, what happens, and for how long. The doctor can locate a sample and grant the exceptional antiepileptic drug to help.

You might also find it helpful to wear a medical alert bracelet with records about the AED pills you use (or shouldn't use).

Coping With Bodily Facet Outcomes

Common bodily aspects results from every remedy choice for a brain tumor are indexed withinside the Types of Treatment phase. Learn extra approximate outcomes of a brain tumor and its remedy, together with methods to save you or manage them. Changes for your bodily fitness rely upon numerous factors, which includes the tumor's vicinity and grade, the duration and dose of remedy, and your standard fitness.

Talk together with your fitness care group often about how you're feeling. It is critical to allow them to recognize approximately any new facet results or adjustments in present facet results. If they recognise how you're feeling, they are able to discover methods to alleviate or manipulate your aspect consequences that will help you experience extra snug and probably preserve any aspect consequences from worsening.

You might also additionally discover it useful to hold a song of your aspect consequences so it's far simpler to provide an explanation for any modifications together with your fitness care group. Learn extra about why monitoring facet results is useful.

Sometimes, aspect consequences can remain after the remedy ends. Doctors name those long-time period aspect results. They name aspect results that arise months or years after remedy past due outcomes. Treating long-time period facet outcomes and past due outcomes is an essential part of survivorship care. Learn extra through analyzing the Follow-up Care segment of this manual or speaking together along with your physician.

Coping With Emotional And Social Outcomes
You will have emotional and social outcomes after a brain tumor diagnosis. This may also consist of coping with loads of emotions, including sadness, tension, or anger, or handling your pressure level. Sometimes, humans locate it tough to specific how they experience to their cherished ones. Some have discovered that

speaking to an oncology social worker, counselor, or member of the clergy can assist them broaden extra powerful methods of coping and support for a brain tumor.

Patients and their households are advocated to percentage their emotions with a member in their fitness care group. You also can discover coping techniques for emotional and social outcomes in a separate segment of this website. This segment consists of many sources for locating assist and data to fulfill your needs.

Coping With The Charges Of Most Cancers Care

Treatment for a brain tumor may be expensive. It can be a supply of strain and tension for sufferers and their households. In addition to remedy expenses, many humans locate they have got extra, unplanned costs associated with their care. For a few humans, the excessive price of hospital treatment stops them from following or finishing their remedy plan. This can position their fitness at threat and might cause better fees withinside the future. Patients and their households are advocated to speak about monetary worries with a member in their fitness care group. Learn more about dealing with monetary concerns in a separate part of this website.

Coping With Obstacles To Care

Different corporations of humans enjoy exceptional fees of the latest most cancers instances and enjoy extraordinary results from their most cancers. These variations are referred to as "most cancer disparities." Disparities are brought about in component through real-global obstacles to great hospital therapy and extra regularly negatively have an effect on racial and ethnic minorities, negative humans, sexual and gender minorities (LGBTQ), adolescent and younger person populations, older adults, and those who stay in rural regions or different underserved communities.

If you're having problems getting the care you want, communicate with a member of your fitness care crew or discover different assets that assist medically underserved humans.

Caring For A Cherished One With A Brain Tumor

Family individuals and pals frequently play an essential position in looking after someone with a brain tumor. This is known as being a caregiver. Caregivers can offer bodily, practical, and emotional guidance to the patient, although they stay a long way away. Being a caregiver also can be annoying and emotionally challenging. One of the maximum critical duties for caregivers is being concerned for themselves.

Patients with a brain tumor frequently want a variety of guides at home. Many sufferers won't be capable of doing sports vital for his or her care, which includes using to and from appointments. And a few might also additionally want changed residing preparations to deal with bodily challenges. This way that caregivers have a variety of obligations on a day by day or as-wished basis, consisting of:

- Providing guide and encouragement
- Talking with the fitness care group
- Giving medications
- Helping manipulate signs and facet results of the tumor and remedy
- Coordinating clinical appointments
- Providing transportation
- Assisting with meals
- Helping with family chores
- Handling coverage and billing issues

Anticipating modifications in mood, personality, and questioning and understanding the way to high-satisfactory address those adjustments

A caregiving plan can assist caregivers live prepared and assist pick out possibilities to delegate duties to others. It can be useful to invite the fitness care group how a good deal of care could be wanted at home and with each day responsibilities at some stage in and after remedy. Use this 1-web page truth sheet to assist make a caregiving movement plan. This loose truth sheet is to be had as a PDF, so it is straightforward to print.

Learn extra approximately caregiving or examine the ASCO Answers Guide to Caring for a Loved One in English or Spanish.

Talking Together Along With Your Fitness Care Crew Approximately Facet Results

Before beginning to remedy, communicate together along with your health practitioner approximately viable aspects. Ask:

- Which aspect outcomes are maximum probably?
- When are they possible?
- What are we able to do to save you or relieve them?

Be positive to inform your fitness care crew approximately any aspect outcomes that occur for the duration of remedy and afterward, too. Tell them even in case you now no longer assume the facet outcomes are serious. This dialogue has to encompass bodily, emotional, social, and monetary consequences.

CONCLUSION

With a little help, most humans can research to manage their emotions and the adjustments brought on by a brain tumor and its treatment. Brain surgical treatment is a lot for your physique to cope with. You can learn how to reap extra manipulation each step of the way. This is true for both sufferers and the humans who care for them.

- It's normal to feel scared, insecure, stressed, and angry about a brain tumor diagnosis– and it is possible to deal with these feelings.
- Try to be an affected person with yourself, your loved ones, and the very slow-moving remedy process.
- You can take an empowerment strategy to attain a sense of management over this disease.

- No query is wrong to ask.
- Take time to procedure the information you're given. You possibly have enough time to take a deep breath and assume about your next steps.
- Talk brazenly with your household and your physicians to help keep the therapy system on target.
- Aim to experience the things that make your life special.

Care for Yourself - Things to Remember

- You can assist your loved one to assume via remedy options, goals, and priorities for the duration of this hard period.
- The medical group can help you know what to expect and how to plan. Recovery after a cure can take time, and it helps to be prepared. Ask all of your questions.
- You can get suggestions from humans who are additionally caring for any

individual with a brain tumor. These people are often very helpful.

- You can ask for help, and say "YES!" when anybody offers. Your well-being needs to ask for and take delivery of help. Online organizers (like MyLifeLine.org) can be very useful.

- Schedule self-care into your day. You can't help others unless you take care of your physical, economic, religious, and emotional well-being.

- End-of-life care plans can help your cherished one sense greater control. Try to get key household contributors to speak about plans. Make positive the medical doctor is conscious of your loved one's preferences.

- If you are grieving the existence you used to know, it's normal. Give yourself time to grieve.

- Focus on the matters that sincerely matter. Find approaches to enjoy the little moments together.

When a Loved One's Personality Changes
Depression, anger, confusion, and temper swings
are frequent signs and symptoms for people with
brain tumors. Personality swings are caused by
the tumor, the treatment, or the patient has run
out of ways to cope. In all cases, these
adjustments can be very hard to manage,
whether or not they are small or drastic.

Speak with your physician if you word these
types of changes. Many emotional shifts can be
treated.

Tips To Manage Difficult Moments

- Don't let your personal feelings of anger,
  resentment, or guilt grow. Admit your
  feelings so you can address the problem.
- Be compassionate with yourself. There's
  no one way a caregiver ought to feel.
  Permit yourself to separate your feelings
  from your actions.

- Ask your assistant community for some coping ideas. Call a family assembly and say, "Let's discern out how we can help each other."

- Set limits. It's k to say "no" when you can't do something.

- Remember that you do not want to have all the answers or restore all the problems.

- Often, simply "being there" and quietly listening is all that's needed. Listen, but strive now not to react to irrational behavior.

Making Important Decisions

Often, a brain tumor will make it tougher to actually think and method information. This may additionally be from the tumor urgent on the brain, from treatment, or from commonly feeling overwhelmed. Whatever the cause, a cherished one may additionally have to emerge as the patient's advocate and care coordinator. If you should be the therapy decision-maker, consider that you can take time to ask questions, research options, and locate support.

Brain tumors are now not identical to different major life events. They can be ongoing and often unpredictable. Try to think through sensible short- and long-term expectations.

Tips for Making Important Decisions

- Learn about the brain tumor's type, location, grade, remedy options, and expectations for restoration and aspect effects.
- Talk to the first-class professionals you can find in your loved one's (or you're) place for a first and 2nd opinion.
- Research credible websites, like the National Cancer Institute, and the National Brain Tumor Society.
- Weigh the professionals and cons of every therapy choice with your cherished one. This ought to consist of things like time, region, and cost.

- Create a "to-do" list of short and long-term needs. Decide what your cherished one can do with and barring help.
- Recognize and respect the competencies and desires of your cherished one.
- Set limits for yourself. Define what you can and can't do for your cherished one.
- Organize a care plan with others. Stress open communication. (Who is doing what, and when?). This plan will assist decrease household stress and bring wished relief.
- Remember that every stage of care calls for extraordinary tiers of support. Roles will trade along the way.
- Gather copies of medical and cure documents (including operation reviews and x-rays). If it makes sense, ask to be the criminal "Power of Attorney" for your cherished one so you can assist with follow-up care plans and future scientific decisions.
- Talk to an oncology social worker at the most cancers middle or with your

oncologist. They can reply to many logistical, non-public, and financial questions.
- Try to price the accurate moments you spend with your cherished one. Every moment is special.

Moving Forward

It's horrifying to envision an exceptional future than you planned. It can additionally be hard to speak about painful topics.

Finding ways to speak about what is taking place makes most human beings experience relief. The conversation often leads to hope about the lifestyles you have collectively now. Often, humans choose to make the most of their time together with family, as they make peace with the circumstance. These can be uplifting conversations that supply you with a feeling of peace.

www.ingramcontent.com/pod-product-compliance
Lightning Source LLC
Chambersburg PA
CBHW052113150726
48002CB00006B/2337